The Vegan Cookbook Made Easy

Made Simple Cookbook with Quick, Easy and Healthy Vegan Recipes for Everyday Cooking and Increase your Mood!

Augustine Johns

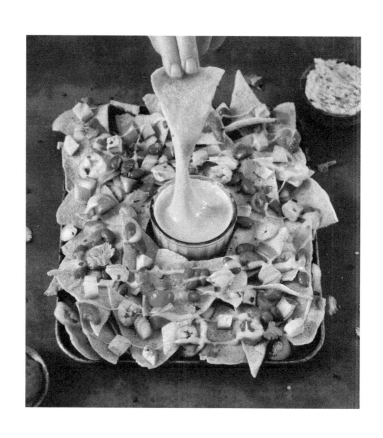

Table of Contents

The information in the following pages is broadly considered a truthful and accurate account of facts and as such, any inattention, use, or misuse of the information in question by the reader will render any resulting actions solely under their purview. There are no scenarios in which the publisher or the original author of this work can be in any fashion deemed liable for any hardship or damages that may befall them after undertaking information described herein.

Additionally, the information in the following pages is intended only for informational purposes and should thus be thought of as universal. As befitting its nature, it is presented without assurance regarding its prolonged validity or interim quality. Trademarks that are mentioned are done without written consent and can in no way be considered an endorsement from the trademark holder.

INTRODUCTION

The Merriam Webster Dictionary defines a vegetarian as one contains a wholly of vegetables, grains, nuts, fruits, and sometimes eggs or dairy products. It has also been described as a plant-based diet that relies wholly on plant-foods such as fruits, whole grains, herbs, vegetables, nuts, seeds, and spices. Whatever way you want to look at it, the reliance wholly on plants stands the vegetarian diet out from other types of diets. People become vegetarians for different reasons. Some take up this nutritional plan for medical or health reasons. For example, people suffering from cardiovascular diseases or who stand the risk of developing such diseases are usually advised to refrain from meat generally and focus on a plant-based diet, rich in fruits and vegetables. Some other individuals become vegetarians for religious or ethical reasons.

On this side of the spectrum are Hinduism, Jainism, Buddhism, Seventh-Day Adventists, and some other religions. It is believed that being a vegetarian is part of being holy and keeping with the ideals of non-violence. For ethical reasons, some animal rights activists are also vegetarians based on the belief that animals have rights and should not be slaughtered for food. Yet another set of persons become vegetarians based on food preference. Such individuals are naturally more disposed to a plant-based diet and find meat and other related food products less pleasurable. Some refrain from meat as a protest against climate change. This is based on the environmental concern that rearing livestock contributes to climate change and greenhouse gas emissions and the waste of natural resources in maintaining such livestock. People are usually very quick to throw words around without exactly knowing what a Vegetarian Diet means. In the same vein, the term "vegetarian" has become a popular one in recent years. What exactly does this word connote, and what does it not mean?

At its simplest, the word "vegetarian" refers to a person who refrains from eating meat, beef, pork, lard, chicken, or even fish. Depending on the kind of vegetarian it is, however, a vegetarian could either eat or exclude from his diet animal products. Animal products would refer to foods such as eggs, dairy products, and even honey! A vegetarian diet would, therefore, refer to the nutritional plan of the void of meat. It is the eating lifestyle of individuals who depend on plant-based foods for nutrition. It excludes animal products, particularly meat - a common denominator for all kinds of Vegetarians - from their diets. A vegetarian could also be defined as a meal plan that consists of foods coming majorly from plants to the exclusion of meat, poultry, and seafood.

This kind of Vegetarian diet usually contains no animal protein.

It is completely understandable from the discussion so far that the term "vegetarian" is more or less a blanket term covering different plant-based diets. While reliance majorly on plant foods is consistent in all the different types of vegetarians, they have some underlying differences. The different types of vegetarians are discussed below:

Veganism: This is undoubtedly the strictest type of vegetarian diet. Vegans exclude the any animal product. It goes as far as avoiding animal-derived ingredients contained in processed foods. Whether its meat, poultry products like eggs, dairy products inclusive of milk, honey, or even gelatin, they all are excluded from the vegans.

Some vegans go beyond nutrition and go as far as refusing to wear clothes that contain animal products. This means such vegans do not wear leather, wool, or silk.

Lacto-vegetarian: This kind of vegetarian excludes meat, fish, and poultry. However, it allows the inclusion of dairy products such as milk, yogurt, cheese, and butter. The hint is perhaps in the name since Lacto means milk in Latin.

Ovo-Vegetarian: Meat and dairy products are excluded under this diet, but eggs could be consumed. Ovo means egg.

Lacto-Ovo Vegetarian: This appears to be the hybrid of the Ovo Vegetarian and the Lacto-Vegetarian. This is the most famous type of vegetarian diet and is usually what comes to mind when people think of the Vegetarian. This type of Vegetarian bars all kinds of meat but allows for the consumption of eggs and dairy products.

Pollotarian: This vegetarian allows the consumption of chicken.

Pescatarian: This refers to the vegetarian that consumes fish. More people are beginning to subscribe to this kind of diet due to health reasons.

Flexitarian: Flexitarians are individuals who prefer plant-based foods to meat but have no problem eating meats once in a while. They are also referred to as semi-vegetarians.

Raw Vegan: This is also called the raw food and consists of a vegan that is yet to be processed and has also not been heated over 46 C. This kind of diet has its root in the belief that nutrients and minerals present in the plant diet are lost when cooked on temperature above 46 C and could also become harmful to the body.

Smoky Red Beans and Rice

Preparation Time: 15 minutes

Cooking Time: 6 minutes

Servings: 6

Ingredients:

- 30 ounce of cooked red beans
- 1 cup of brown rice, uncooked
- 1 cup of chopped green pepper
- 1 cup of chopped celery
- 1 cup of chopped white onion
- 1 1/2 teaspoon of minced garlic
- 1/2 teaspoon of salt
- 1/4 teaspoon of cayenne pepper
- 1 teaspoon of smoked paprika
- 2 teaspoons of dried thyme
- 1 bay leaf
- 2 1/3 cups of vegetable broth

Directions:

1. Using a 6-quarts slow cooker, place all the ingredients except for the rice, salt, and cayenne pepper.

2. Stir until it mixes properly and then cover the top.

3. Plug in the slow cooker, adjust the cooking time to 4 hours, and steam on a low heat setting.

4. Then pour in and stir the rice, salt, cayenne pepper and continue cooking for an additional 2 hours at a high heat setting.

5. Serve straight away.

Nutrition: Calories: 791 kcal Protein: 3.25 g Fat: 86.45 g Carbohydrates: 9.67 g

Spicy Black-Eyed Peas

Preparation Time: 12 minutes

Cooking Time: 8 hours and 8 minutes

Servings: 8

Ingredients:

- 32-ounce black-eyed peas, uncooked
- 1 cup of chopped orange bell pepper
- 1 cup of chopped celery
- 8-ounce of chipotle peppers, chopped
- 1 cup of chopped carrot
- 1 cup of chopped white onion
- 1 teaspoon of minced garlic
- 3/4 teaspoon of salt
- 1/2 teaspoon of ground black pepper
- 2 teaspoons of liquid smoke flavoring
- 2 teaspoons of ground cumin
- 1 tablespoon of adobo sauce
- 2 tablespoons of olive oil
- 1 tablespoon of apple cider vinegar
- 4 cups of vegetable broth

Directions:

1. Place a medium-sized non-stick skillet pan over an average temperature of heat; add the bell peppers, carrot, onion, garlic, oil, and vinegar.
2. Stir until it mixes properly and let it cook for 5 to 8 minutes or until it gets translucent.
3. Transfer this mixture to a 6-quarts slow cooker and add the peas, chipotle pepper, adobo sauce, and the vegetable broth.
4. Stir until mixed properly and cover the top.
5. Plug in the slow cooker, adjust the cooking time to 8 hours, and let it cook on the low heat setting or until peas are soft.
6. Serve right away.

Nutrition: Calories: 1071 kcal Protein: 5.3 g Fat: 113.65 g Carbohydrates: 18.51 g

Creamy Artichoke Soup

Preparation Time: 5 minutes

Cooking Time: 40 minutes

Servings: 4

Ingredients:

- 1 can artichoke hearts, drained
- 3 cups vegetable broth
- 2 tbsp. lemon juice
- 1 small onion, finely cut
- 2 cloves garlic, crushed
- 3 tbsp. olive oil
- 2 tbsp. flour
- ½ cup vegan cream

Directions:

1. Gently sauté the onion and garlic in some olive oil. Add the flour, whisking constantly, and then add the hot vegetable broth slowly, while still whisking. Cook for about 5 minutes.

2. Blend the artichoke, lemon juice, salt, and pepper until smooth. Add the puree to the broth mix, stir well, and then stir in the cream. Cook

until heated through. Garnish with a swirl of vegan cream or a sliver of artichoke.

Nutrition: Calories: 1622 kcal Protein: 4.45 g Fat: 181.08 g Carbohydrates: 10.99 g

Tomato Artichoke Soup

Preparation Time: 5 minutes

Cooking Time: 35 minutes

Servings: 4

Ingredients:

- 1 can artichoke hearts, drained
- 1 can diced tomatoes, undrained
- 3 cups vegetable broth
- 1 small onion, chopped
- 2 cloves garlic, crushed
- 1 tbsp. pesto
- Black pepper, to taste

Directions:

1. Combine all ingredients in the slow cooker.
2. Cover and cook on low for 8-10 hours or on high for 4-5 hours.
3. Blend the soup in batches then put it back to the slow cooker. Season with pepper and salt, then serve.

Nutrition: Calories: 1487 kcal Protein: 3.98 g Fat: 167.42 g Carbohydrates: 8.2 g

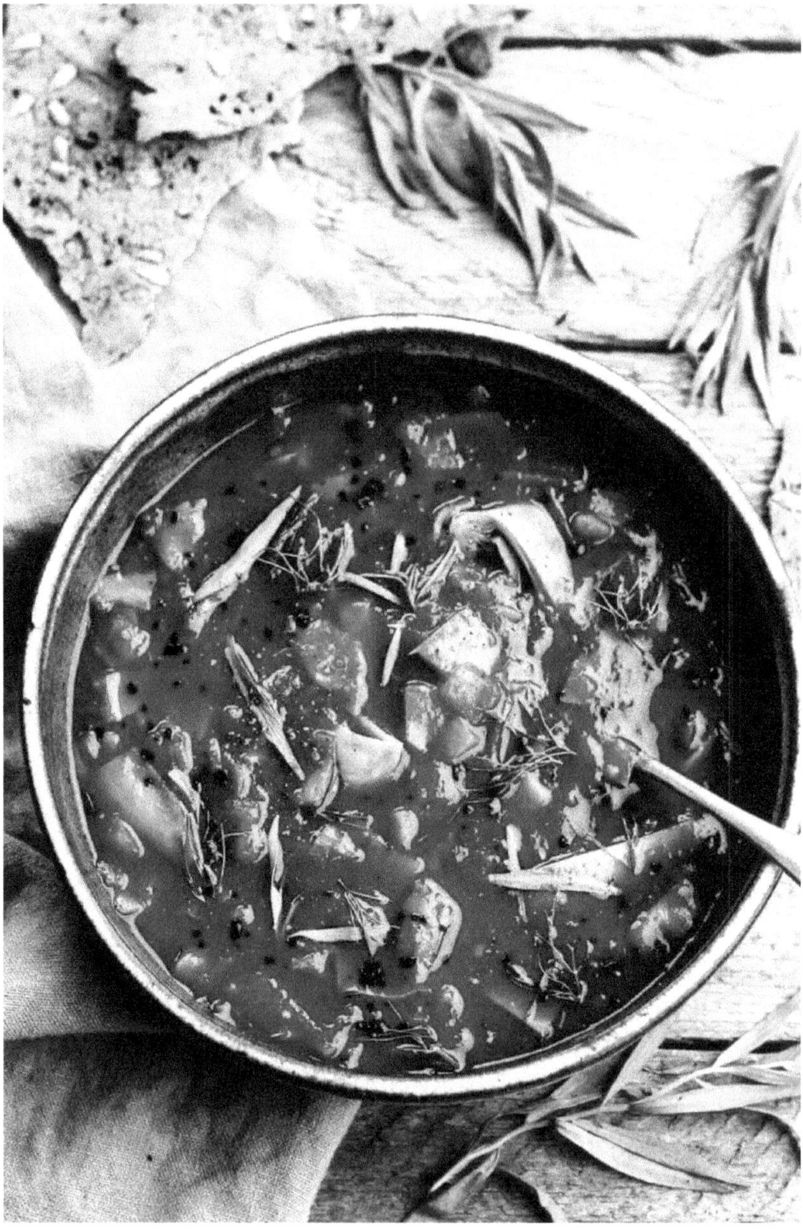

Super Radish Avocado Salad

Preparation Time: 10 minutes

Cooking Time: 25 minutes

Servings: 2

Ingredients:

- 6 shredded carrots
- 6 ounces diced radishes
- 1 diced avocado
- 1/3 cup ponzu

Directions:

1. Place all together the ingredients in a serving bowl and toss. Enjoy!

Nutrition: Calories: 292 Kcal Protein: 7.42 g Fat: 18.29 g Carbohydrates: 29.59 g

Beauty School Ginger Cucumbers

Preparation Time: 10 minutes

Cooking Time: 45 minutes

Servings: 14

Ingredients:

- 1 sliced cucumber
- 3 tsp. rice wine vinegar
- 1 ½ tbsp. sugar
- 1 tsp. minced ginger

Directions:

1. Place all together the ingredients in a mixing bowl, and toss the ingredients well. Enjoy!

Nutrition: Calories: 10 kcal Protein: 0.46 g Fat: 0.43 g Carbohydrates: 0.89 g

Exotic Butternut Squash and Chickpea Curry

Preparation Time: 20 minutes

Cooking Time: 6 hours

Servings: 8

Ingredients:

- 1 1/2 cups of shelled peas
- 1 1/2 cups of chickpeas, uncooked and rinsed
- 2 1/2 cups of diced butternut squash
- 12 ounce of chopped spinach
- 2 large tomatoes, diced
- 1 small white onion, peeled and chopped
- 1 teaspoon of minced garlic
- 1 teaspoon of salt
- 3 tablespoons of curry powder
- 14-ounce of coconut milk
- 3 cups of vegetable broth
- 1/4 cup of chopped cilantro

Directions:

1. Using a 6-quarts slow cooker, place all the ingredients into it except for the spinach and peas.

2. Cover the top, plug in the slow cooker; adjust the cooking time to 6 hours, and cook on the high heat setting or until the chickpeas get tender.

3. 30 minutes to ending your cooking, add the peas and spinach to the slow cooker and cook for the remaining 30 minutes.

4. Stir to check the sauce; if the sauce is runny, stir in a mixture of a 1 tbsp. Cornstarch mixed with 2 tbsp. Water.

5. Serve with boiled rice.

Nutrition: Calories: 774 kcal Protein: 3.71 g Fat: 83.25 g Carbohydrates: 12.64 g

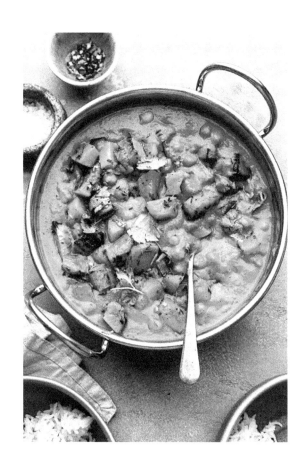

Sage Walnuts and Radishes

Preparation Time: 10 minutes

Cooking Time: 10 minutes

Servings: 6

Ingredients:

- 2 tablespoons olive oil
- 5 celery ribs, chopped
- 3 spring onions, chopped
- ½ pound radishes, halved
- juice of 1 lime
- Zest of 1 lime, grated
- 8 ounces walnuts, chopped
- A pinch of black pepper
- 3 tablespoons sage, chopped

Directions:

1. Heat up a pan with the oil over medium heat, add celery and spring onion, stir and cook for 5 minutes.
2. Add the rest of the ingredients, toss, cook for another 5 minutes, divide into bowls and serve.

Nutrition: Calories 200 Fat 7 Fiber 5 Carbs 9.3

Protein 4

Chili Fennel

Preparation Time: 10 minutes

Cooking Time: 8 minutes

Servings: 4

Ingredients:

- 2 fennel bulbs, cut into quarters
- 3 tablespoons olive oil
- Salt and black pepper to the taste
- 1 garlic clove, minced
- 1 red chili pepper, chopped
- ¾ cup veggie stock
- Juice of ½ lemon

Directions:

1. Heat a pan that fits your Air Fryer with the oil over medium-high heat, add garlic and chili pepper, stir and cook for 2 minutes.
2. Add fennel, salt, pepper, stock, and lemon juice, toss to coat, introduce in your Air Fryer and cook at 350 ° F for at least 6 minutes.
3. Divide into plates and serve as a side dish.

Nutrition: Calories: 158 kcal Protein: 3.57 g Fat: 11.94 g Carbohydrates: 11.33 g

Collard Greens and Tomatoes

Preparation Time: 10 minutes

Cooking Time: 10 minutes

Servings: 9

Ingredients:

- 1 pound collard greens
- ¼ cup cherry tomatoes, halved
- 1 tablespoon apple cider vinegar
- 2 tablespoons veggie stock
- Salt and black pepper to the taste

Directions:

1. In a pan that fits the Air Fryer, combine tomatoes, collard greens, vinegar, stock, salt, and pepper, stir, introduce in your Air Fryer and cook at 320 ° F for 10 minutes.

2. Divide between plates and serve as a side dish.

Nutrition: Calories: 28 kcal Protein: 2.34 g Fat: 0.99 g Carbohydrates: 3.26 g

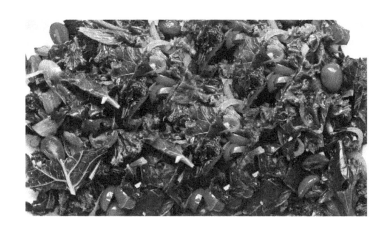

Bean and Carrot Spirals

Preparation Time: 10 minutes

Cooking Time: 40 minutes

Servings: 24

Ingredients:

- 4 8-inch flour tortillas
- 1 ½ cups of Easy Mean White Bean dip
- 10 ounces spinach leaves
- ½ cup diced carrots
- ½ cup diced red peppers

Directions:

1. Starts by preparing the bean dip, seen above. Next, spread out the bean dip on each tortilla, making sure to leave about a ¾ inch white border on the tortillas' surface. Next, place spinach in the center of the tortilla, followed by carrots and red peppers.
2. Roll the tortillas into tight rolls, and cover every rolls with plastic wrap or aluminum foil.
3. Let them chill in the fridge for twenty-four hours.

4. Afterward, remove the wrap from the spirals and remove the very ends of the rolls. Slice the rolls into six individual spiral pieces, and arrange them on a platter for serving. Enjoy!

Nutrition: Calories: 205 kcal Protein: 6.41 g Fat: 4.16 g Carbohydrates: 35.13 g

Tofu Nuggets with Barbecue Glaze

Preparation Time: 10 minutes

Cooking Time: 25 minutes

Servings: 9

Ingredients:

- 32 ounces tofu
- 1 cup quick vegan barbecue sauce

Directions:

1. Set the oven to 425F.
2. Next, slice the tofu and blot the tofu with clean towels. Next, slice and dice the tofu and completely eliminate the water from the tofu material.
3. Stir the tofu with the vegan barbecue sauce, and place the tofu on a baking sheet.
4. Bake the tofu for fifteen minutes. Afterward, stir the tofu and bake the tofu for an additional ten minutes.
5. Enjoy!

Nutrition: Calories: 311 kcal Protein: 19.94 g
Fat: 21.02 g Carbohydrates: 15.55 g

Peppered Pinto Beans

Preparation Time: 10 minutes

Cooking Time: 15 minutes

Servings: 6

Ingredients:

- 1 tsp. Chili powder
- 1 tsp. ground cumin
- .5 cup Vegetable
- 2 cans Pinto beans
- 1 Minced jalapeno
- 1 Diced red bell pepper
- 1 tsp. Olive oil

Directions:

1. Take out a pot and heat the oil. Cook the jalapeno and pepper for a bit before adding in the pepper, salt, cumin, broth, and beans.
2. Place to a boil and then reduce the heat to cook for a bit. After 10 minutes, let it cool and serve.

Nutrition: Calories: 183 Carbs: 32g Fat: 2g Protein: 11g

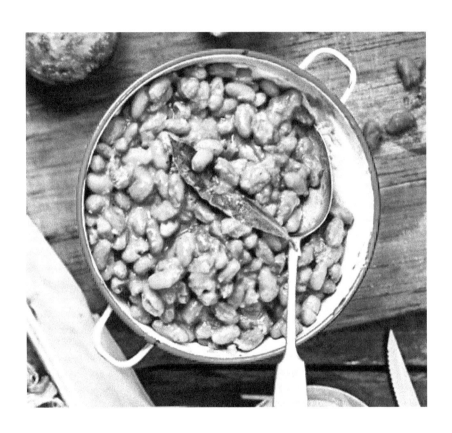

Black Bean Pizza

Preparation Time: 30 minutes

Cooking Time: 20 minutes

Servings: 2

Ingredients:

- 1 Sliced avocado
- 1 Sliced red onion
- 1 Grated carrot
- 1 Sliced tomato
- .5 cup Spicy black bean dip
- 2 Pizza crusts

Directions:

1. Turn on the oven and let heat to 400 degrees. Layout two crusts on a baking sheet and add the dip onto each one.
2. Top with the tomato slices and sprinkle the carrots and the onion on a well.
3. Add to the oven and let it bake for about 20 minutes or so until done. Top with the avocado before serving.

Nutrition: Calories: 379 Carbs: 59g Fat: 13g

Protein: 13g

Vegetable and Chickpea Loaf

Preparation Time: 10 minutes

Cooking Time: 15 minutes

Servings: 4

Ingredients:

- 1 tsp. Salt
- .5 tsp. Dried sage
- 1 tsp. Dried savory
- 1 tbsp. Soy sauce
- .25 cup Parsley
- .5 cup Breadcrumbs
- .75 cup Oats
- .75 cup Chickpea flour
- 1.5 cup cooked chickpeas
- 2 Minced garlic cloves
- 1 Chopped yellow onion
- 1 Shredded carrot
- 1 Shredded white potato

Directions:

1. Set the oven to 350F. Take out a loaf pan and then grease it up.

2. Squeeze out the liquid from the potato and add to the food processor with the garlic, onion, and carrot.

3. Add the chickpeas and pulse to blend well. Add in the rest of the ingredients here, and when it is done, use your hands to form this into a loaf and add to the pan.

4. Place into the oven to bake for a bit until it is nice and firm. Let it cool down and then slice.

Nutrition: Calories: 351 kcal Protein: 16.86 g Fat: 6.51 g Carbohydrates: 64 g

Thyme and Lemon Couscous

Preparation Time: 5 minutes

Cooking Time: 10 minutes

Servings: 6

Ingredients:

- .25 cup Chopped parsley
- 1.5 cup Couscous
- 2 tbsp. Chopped thyme
- Juice and zest of a lemon
- 2.75 cup Vegetable stock

Directions:

1. Take out a pot and add in the thyme, lemon juice, and vegetable stock. Stir in the couscous after it has gotten to a boil and then take off the heat.
2. Allow sitting covered until it can take in all of the liquid. Then fluff up with a form.
3. Stir in the parsley and lemon zest, then serve warm.

Nutrition: Calories: 922 kcal Protein: 2.7 g Fat: 101.04 g Carbohydrates: 10.02 g

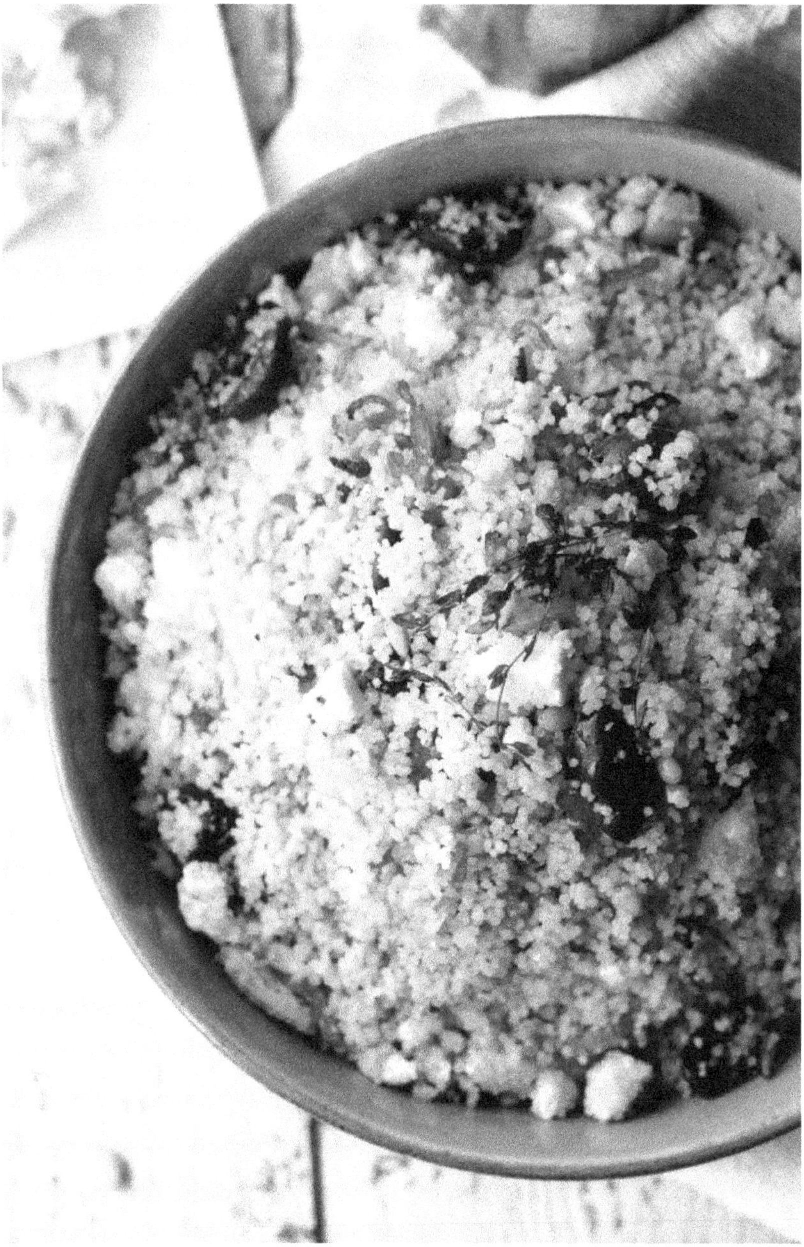

Pesto and White Bean Pasta

Preparation Time: 10 minutes

Cooking Time: 10 minutes

Servings: 4

Ingredients:

- .5 cup Chopped black olives
- .25 Diced red onion
- 1 cup Chopped tomato
- .5 cup Spinach pesto
- 1.5 cup Cannellini beans
- 8 oz. Rotini pasta, cooked

Directions:

1. Bring out a bowl and toss together the pesto, beans, and pasta.
2. Add in the olives, red onion, and tomato and toss around a bit more before serving.

Nutrition: Calories 544 Carbs 83g Fat 17g Protein 23g

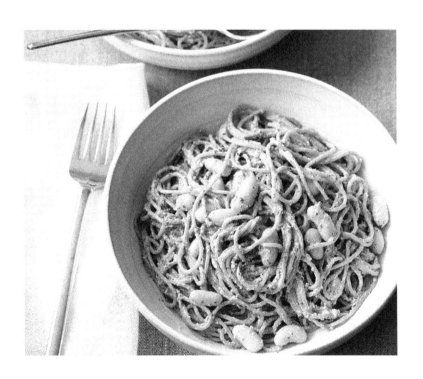

Baked Okra and Tomato

Preparation Time: 10 minutes

Cooking Time: 75 minutes

Servings: 6

Ingredients:

- ½ cup lima beans, frozen
- 4 tomatoes, chopped
- 8 ounces okra, fresh and washed, stemmed, sliced into ½ inch thick slices
- 1 onion, sliced into rings
- ½ sweet pepper, seeded and sliced thin
- Pinch of crushed red pepper
- Salt to taste

Directions:

1. Preheat your oven to 350 degrees Fahrenheit
2. Cook lima beans in water accordingly and drain them, take a 2quart casserole tin
3. Add all listed ingredients to the dish and cover with foil, bake for 45 minutes
4. Uncover the dish, stir well and bake for 35 minutes more

5. Stir then serve, and enjoy!

Nutrition: Calories: 55 Fat: 0g Carbohydrates: 12g Protein: 3g

Curried Apple

Preparation Time: 10 minutes

Cooking Time: 90 minutes

Servings: 4

Ingredients:

- 1 tablespoon fresh lemon juice
- ½ cup of water
- 2 apples, Fuji or Honeycrisp, cored and thinly sliced into rings
- 1 teaspoon curry powder

Directions:

1. Set the oven to 200F, take a rimmed baking sheet and line with parchment paper
2. Take a bowl and mix in lemon juice and water, add apples and soak for 2 minutes
3. Pat them dry and arrange in a single layer on your baking sheet, dust curry powder on top of apple slices
4. Bake for 45 minutes. After 45 minutes, turn the apples and bake for 45 minutes more

5. Let them cool for extra crispiness, serve and enjoy!

Nutrition: Calories: 240 Fat: 13g Carbohydrates: 20g Protein: 6g

Wild Rice and Millet Croquettes

Preparation Time: 5 minutes

Cooking Time: 20 minutes

Servings: 4

Ingredients:

- ¾ cooked millet
- ½ cup cooked wild rice
- 3 tablespoons extra virgin olive oil
- ¼ cup onion, minced
- 1 celery rib, finely minced
- ¼ cup carrot, shredded
- 1/3 cup all-purpose flour
- ¼ cup fresh parsley, chopped
- 2 teaspoons dried dill weed
- Salt and pepper to taste

Directions:

1. Add cooked millet and wild rice to a large-sized bowl, keep it to one side
2. Take a medium skillet and add 1 tablespoon of oil, place it over medium heat

3. Put onion, celery, and carrot and cook for at least 5 minutes
4. Add veggies and stir in flour, parsley, salt, pepper, and dill weed
5. Mix well and transfer to the fridge, let it sit for 20 minutes
6. Use hands to shape mixture into small patties, take a large skillet and place it over medium heat
7. Add 2 tablespoons of oil and let it heat up
8. Add croquettes and cook for 8 minutes in total until golden brown
9. Serve and enjoy!

Nutrition: Calories: 250 Fat: 9g Carbohydrates: 33g Protein: 9g

Grilled Eggplant Steaks

Preparation Time: 10 minutes

Cooking Time: 10 minutes

Servings: 4

Ingredients:

- 4 Roma tomatoes, diced
- 8 ounces cashew cream
- 2 eggplants
- 1 tablespoon olive oil
- 1 cup parsley, chopped
- 1 cucumber, diced
- Salt and pepper to taste

Directions:

1. Slice eggplants into three thick steaks, drizzle with oil, and season with salt and pepper
2. Grill in a pan for 4 minutes per side
3. Top with remaining ingredients
4. Serve and enjoy!

Nutrition: Calories: 86 Fat: 7g Carbohydrates: 12g Protein: 8g

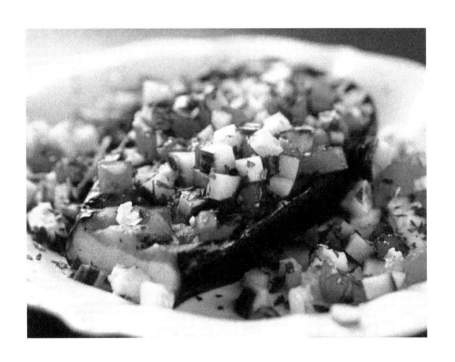

Steamed Cauliflower

Preparation Time: 5 minutes

Cooking Time: 10 minutes

Servings: 6

Ingredients:

- 1 large head cauliflower
- 1 cup water
- ½ teaspoon salt
- 1 teaspoon red pepper flakes (optional)

Directions:

1. Remove any leaves from the cauliflower, and cut it into florets.
2. In a large saucepan, bring the water to a boil. Place a steamer basket over the water, and add the florets and salt. Cover and steam for 5 to 7 minutes, until tender.
3. In a large bowl, toss the cauliflower with the red pepper flakes (if using). Transfer the florets to a large airtight container or 6 single-serving containers. Let cool before sealing the lids.

Nutrition: Calories: 35 Fat: 0g Protein: 3g Carbohydrates: 7g Fiber: 4g Sugar: 4g Sodium: 236mg

Cajun Sweet Potatoes

Preparation Time: 5 minutes

Cooking Time: 30 minutes

Servings: 4

Ingredients:

- 2 pounds sweet potatoes
- 2 teaspoons extra-virgin olive oil
- ½ teaspoon ground cayenne pepper
- ½ teaspoon smoked paprika
- ½ teaspoon dried oregano
- ½ teaspoon dried thyme
- ½ teaspoon garlic powder
- ½ teaspoon salt (optional)

Directions:

1. Preheat the oven to 400ºF. Line a baking sheet with parchment paper.
2. Wash the potatoes, pat dry, and cut into ¾-inch cubes. Transfer to a large bowl, and pour the olive oil over the potatoes.
3. In a small bowl, combine the cayenne, paprika, oregano, thyme, and garlic powder. Sprinkle the

spices over the potatoes and combine until the potatoes are well coated. Spread the potatoes on the prepared baking sheet in a single layer. Season with the salt (if using). Roast for 30 minutes, stirring the potatoes after 15 minutes.

4. Divide the potatoes evenly among 4 single-serving containers. Let cool completely before sealing.

Nutrition: Calories: 219 Fat: 3g Protein: 4g Carbohydrates: 46g Fiber: 7g Sugar: 9g Sodium: 125mg

Smoky Coleslaw

Preparation Time: 10 minutes

Cooking Time: 0 minute

Servings: 6

Ingredients:

- 1-pound shredded cabbage
- 1/3 cup vegan mayonnaise
- ¼ cup unseasoned rice vinegar
- 3 tablespoons plain vegan yogurt or plain soymilk
- 1 tablespoon vegan sugar
- ½ teaspoon salt
- ¼ teaspoon freshly ground black pepper
- ¼ teaspoon smoked paprika
- ¼ teaspoon chipotle powder

Directions:

1. Put the shredded cabbage in a large bowl. In a medium bowl, whisk the mayonnaise, vinegar, yogurt, sugar, salt, pepper, paprika, and chipotle powder.

2. Pour over the cabbage, and mix with a spoon or spatula and until the cabbage shreds are coated. Divide the coleslaw evenly among 6 single-serving containers. Seal the lids.

Nutrition: Calories: 73 Fat: 4g Protein: 1g Carbohydrates: 8g Fiber: 2g Sugar: 5g Sodium: 283mg

Mediterranean Hummus Pizza

Preparation Time: 10 minutes

Cooking Time: 30 minutes

Servings: 2 pizzas

Ingredients:

- ½ zucchini, thinly sliced
- ½ red onion, thinly sliced
- 1 cup cherry tomatoes, halved
- 2 to 4 tablespoons pitted and chopped black olives
- Pinch sea salt
- Drizzle olive oil (optional)
- 2 prebaked pizza crusts
- ½ cup Classic Hummus
- 2 to 4 tablespoons Cheesy Sprinkle

Directions:

1. Preheat the oven to 400°F. Place the zucchini, onion, cherry tomatoes, and olives in a large bowl, sprinkle them with the sea salt, and toss them a bit. Drizzle with a bit of olive oil (if

using), to seal in the flavor and keep them from drying out in the oven.

2. Lay the two crusts out on a large baking sheet. Spread half the hummus on each crust, and top with the veggie mixture and some Cheesy Sprinkle. Pop the pizzas in the oven for 20 to 30 minutes, or until the veggies are soft.

Nutrition: Calories: 500; Total fat: 25g Carbs: 58g Fiber: 12g Protein:

Baked Brussels Sprouts

Preparation Time: 10 minutes

Cooking Time: 40 minutes

Servings: 4

Ingredients:

- 1-pound Brussels sprouts
- 2 teaspoons extra-virgin olive or canola oil
- 4 teaspoons minced garlic (about 4 cloves)
- 1 teaspoon dried oregano
- ½ teaspoon dried rosemary
- ½ teaspoon salt
- ¼ teaspoon freshly ground black pepper
- 1 tablespoon balsamic vinegar

Directions:

1. Preheat the oven to 400ºF. Line a rimmed baking sheet with parchment paper. Trim and halve the Brussels sprouts. Transfer to a large bowl. Toss with the olive oil, garlic, oregano, rosemary, salt, and pepper to coat well.

2. Transfer to the prepared baking sheet. Bake for 35 to 40 minutes, shaking the pan occasionally

to help with even browning, until crisp on the outside and tender on the inside. Remove from the oven and transfer to a large bowl. Stir in the balsamic vinegar, coating well.

3. Divide the Brussels sprouts evenly among 4 single-serving containers. Let cool before sealing the lids.

Nutrition: Calories: 77 Fat: 3g Protein: 4g Carbohydrates: 12g Fiber: 5g Sugar: 3g Sodium: 320mg

Minted Peas

Preparation Time: 5 minutes

Cooking Time: 5 minutes

Servings: 4

Ingredients:

- 1 tablespoon olive oil
- 4 cups peas, fresh or frozen (not canned)
- ½ teaspoon sea salt
- freshly ground black pepper
- 3 tablespoons chopped fresh mint

Directions:

1. In a large sauté pan, heat the olive oil over medium-high heat until hot. Add the peas and cook, about 5 minutes.
2. Remove the pan from heat. Stir in the salt, season with pepper, and stir in the mint.
3. Serve hot.

Nutrition: Calories: 77 Fat: 3g Protein: 4g Carbohydrates: 12g Fiber: 5g Sugar: 3g Sodium: 320mg

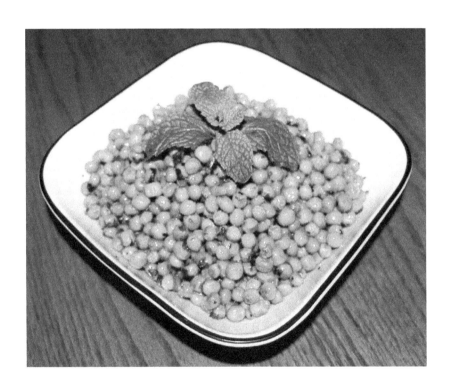

Basic Baked Potatoes

Preparation Time: 5 minutes

Cooking Time: 60 minutes

Servings: 5

Ingredients:

- 5 medium Russet potatoes or a variety of potatoes, washed and patted dry
- 1 to 2 tablespoons extra-virgin olive oil
- ¼ teaspoon salt
- ¼ teaspoon freshly ground black pepper

Directions:

1. Preheat the oven to 400ºF. Pierce each potato several times with a fork or a knife. Brush the olive oil over the potatoes, then rub each with a pinch of the salt and a pinch of the pepper.

2. Place the potatoes on a baking sheet and bake for 50 to 60 minutes, until tender. Place the potatoes on a baking rack and cool completely. Transfer to an airtight container or 5 single-serving containers. Let cool before sealing the lids.

Nutrition: Calories: 171 Fat: 3g Protein: 4g

Carbohydrates: 34g Fiber: 5g Sugar: 3g Sodium:

129mg

Glazed Curried Carrots

Preparation Time: 5 minutes

Cooking Time: 15 minutes

Servings: 6

Ingredients:

- 1-pound carrots, peeled and thinly sliced
- 2 tablespoons olive oil
- 2 tablespoons curry powder
- 2 tablespoons pure maple syrup
- juice of ½ lemon
- sea salt
- freshly ground black pepper

Directions:

1. Place the carrots in a large pot and cover with water. Cook on medium-high heat until tender, about 10 minutes. Drain the carrots and return them to the pan over medium-low heat.

2. Stir in the olive oil, curry powder, maple syrup, and lemon juice. Cook, stirring constantly, until the liquid reduces, about 5 minutes. Season with salt and pepper and serve immediately.

Nutrition: Calories: 171 Fat: 3g Protein: 4g

Carbohydrates: 34g Fiber: 5g Sugar: 3g Sodium:

129mg

Miso Spaghetti Squash

Preparation Time: 5 minutes

Cooking Time: 40 minutes

Servings: 4

Ingredients:

- 1 (3-pound) spaghetti squash
- 1 tablespoon hot water
- 1 tablespoon unseasoned rice vinegar
- 1 tablespoon white miso

Directions:

1. Preheat the oven to 400°F. Line a rimmed baking sheet with parchment paper. Halve the squash lengthwise and place, cut-side down, on the prepared baking sheet.

2. Bake for 35 to 40 minutes, until tender. Cool until the squash is easy to handle. With a fork, scrape out the flesh, which will be stringy, like spaghetti. Transfer to a large bowl. In a small bowl, combine the hot water, vinegar, and miso with a whisk or fork. Pour over the squash. Gently toss with tongs to coat the squash.

3. Divide the squash evenly among 4 single-serving containers. Let cool before sealing the lids.

Nutrition: Calories: 117 Fat: 2g Protein: 3g Carbohydrates: 25g Fiber: 0g Sugar: 0g Sodium: 218mg

Garlic and Herb Noodles

Preparation Time: 10 minutes

Cooking Time: 2 minutes

Servings: 4

Ingredients:

- 1 teaspoon extra-virgin olive oil or 2 tablespoons vegetable broth
- 1 teaspoon minced garlic (about 1 clove)
- 4 medium zucchinis, spiral
- ½ teaspoon dried basil
- ½ teaspoon dried oregano
- ¼ to ½ teaspoon red pepper flakes, to taste
- ¼ teaspoon salt (optional)
- ¼ teaspoon freshly ground black pepper

Directions:

1. In a large skillet over medium-high heat, heat the olive oil.
2. Add the garlic, zucchini, basil, oregano, red pepper flakes, salt (if using), and black pepper. Sauté for 1 to 2 minutes, until barely tender.

Divide the noodles evenly among 4 storage containers. Let cool before sealing the lids.

Nutrition: Calories: 44 Fat: 2g Protein: 3g Carbohydrates: 7g Fiber: 2g Sugar: 3g Sodium: 20mg

Thai Roasted Broccoli

Preparation Time: 5 minutes

Cooking Time: 15 minutes

Servings: 4

Ingredients:

- 1 head broccoli, cut into florets
- 2 tablespoons olive oil
- 1 tablespoon soy sauce or gluten-free tamari

Directions:

1. Preheat the oven to 425°F. Line a baking sheet with parchment paper. In a large bowl, combine the broccoli, oil, and soy sauce. Toss well to combine.
2. Spread the broccoli on the prepared baking sheet. Roast for 10 minutes.
3. Toss the broccoli with a spatula and roast for an additional 5 minutes, or until the edges of the florets begin to brown.

Nutrition: Calories: 44 Fat: 2g Protein: 3g Carbohydrates: 7g Fiber: 2g Sugar: 3g Sodium: 20mg

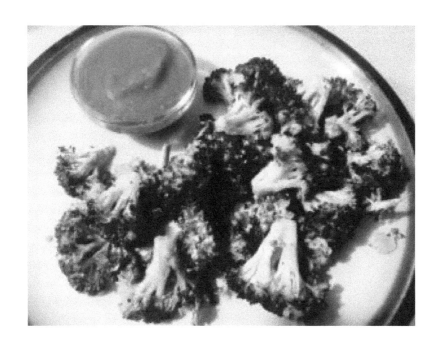

Coconut Curry Noodle

Preparation Time: 10 minutes

Cooking Time: 30 minutes

Servings: 4

Ingredients:

- ½ tablespoon oil
- 3 garlic cloves, minced
- 2 tablespoons lemongrass, minced
- 1 tablespoon fresh ginger, grated
- 2 tablespoons red curry paste
- 1 (14 oz.) can coconut milk
- 1 tablespoon brown sugar
- 2 tablespoons soy sauce
- 2 tablespoons fresh lime juice
- 1 tablespoon hot chili paste
- 12 oz. linguine
- 2 cups broccoli florets
- 1 cup carrots, shredded
- 1 cup edamame, shelled
- 1 red bell pepper, sliced

Directions:

1. Fill a suitably-sizedpot with salted water and boil it on high heat.
2. Add pasta to the boiling water and cook until it is al dente then rinse under cold water.
3. Now place a medium-sized saucepan over medium heat and add oil.
4. Stir in ginger, garlic, and lemongrass, then sauté for 30 seconds.
5. Add coconut milk, soy sauce, curry paste, brown sugar, chili paste, and lime juice.
6. Stir this curry mixture for 10 minutes, or until it thickens.
7. Toss in carrots, broccoli, edamame, bell pepper, and cooked pasta.
8. Mix well, then serve warm.

Nutrition: Calories: 44 Fat: 2g Protein: 3g Carbohydrates: 7g Fiber: 2g Sugar: 3g Sodium: 20mg

Collard Green Pasta

Preparation Time: 10 minutes

Cooking Time: 20 minutes

Servings: 4

Ingredients

- 2 tablespoons olive oil
- 4 garlic cloves, minced
- 8 oz. whole wheat pasta
- ½ cup panko bread crumbs
- 1 tablespoon nutritional yeast
- 1 teaspoon red pepper flakes
- 1 large bunch collard greens
- 1 large lemon, zest and juiced

Directions:

1. Fill a suitable pot with salted water and boil it on high heat.

2. Add pasta to the boiling water and cook until it is al dente, then rinse under cold water.

3. Reserve ½ cup of the cooking liquid from the pasta.

4. Place a non-stick pan over medium heat and add 1 tablespoon olive oil.
5. Stir in half of the garlic, then sauté for 30 seconds.
6. Add breadcrumbs and sauté for approximately 5 minutes.
7. Toss in red pepper flakes and nutritional yeast then mix well.
8. Transfer the breadcrumbs mixture to a plate and clean the pan.
9. Add the remaining tablespoon oil to the nonstick pan.
10. Stir in the garlic clove, salt, black pepper, and chard leaves.
11. Cook for 5 minutes until the leaves are wilted.
12. Add pasta along with the reserved pasta liquid.
13. Mix well, then add garlic crumbs, lemon juice, and zest.
14. Toss well, then serve warm.

Nutrition: Calories: 45 Fat: 2.5g Protein: 4g Carbohydrates: 9g Fiber: 4g Sugar: 3g Sodium: 20mg

DIP AND SPREAD RECIPES

Asparagus Spanakopita

Preparation Time: 25 minutes

Cooking Time: 25 minutes

Servings: 12

Ingredients:

- 2 cups cut fresh asparagus (1-inch pieces)
- 20 sheets phyllo dough, (14 inches x 9 inches)
- Nonstick cooking spray
- Refrigerated butter-flavored spray
- 2 cups torn fresh spinach
- 3 oz. crumbled feta cheese
- 2 tablespoon butter
- 1/4 cup all-purpose flour
- 1-1/2 cups fat-free milk
- 3 tablespoon lemon juice
- 1 teaspoon dill weed
- 1 teaspoon dried thyme
- 1/4 teaspoon salt

Directions:

1. In a steamer basket, put the asparagus and place it on top of a saucepan with 1-inch of water, then boil. Put the cover and let it steam for 5 minutes or until it becomes crisp-tender.

2. Put 1 sheet of phyllo dough in a cooking spray-coated 13x9-inch baking dish, then cut if needed. Use the butter-flavored spray to spritz the dough. Redo the layers 9 times. Lay the asparagus, feta cheese, and spinach on top. Cover it using a sheet of phyllo dough, then spritz it using the butter-flavored spray. Redo the process using the leftover phyllo. Slice it into 12 pieces. Let it bake for 15 minutes at 350 degrees F without cover, or until it turns golden brown.

3. To make the sauce, in a small saucepan, melt the butter. Mix in the flour until it becomes smooth, then slowly add the milk. Stir in salt, thyme, dill, and lemon juice, then boil. Let it cook and stir for 5 minutes until it becomes thick. Serve the spanakopita with the sauce.

Nutrition: Calories 112 Fat 4 Carbs 14 Protein 5

Black Bean and Corn Salsa from Red Gold

Preparation Time: 15 minutes

Cooking Time: 15 minutes

Servings: 25

Ingredients:

- 2 cans black beans, drained and rinsed
- 1 can whole kernel corn, drained
- 2 cans RED GOLD® Petite Diced Tomatoes & Green Chilies
- 1 can RED GOLD® Diced Tomatoes, drained
- 1/2 cup chopped green onions
- 2 tablespoon chopped fresh cilantro
- Salt and black pepper to taste

Directions:

1. Mix all ingredients to combine in a big bowl. Refrigerate to blend flavors for a few hours to overnight. Serve with chips or crackers.

Nutrition: Calories 65 Fat 3 Carbs 8 Protein 9

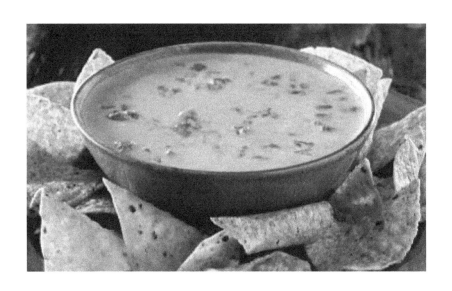

Avocado Bean Dip

Preparation Time: 15 minutes

Cooking Time: 15 minutes

Servings: 2

Ingredients:

- 1 medium ripe avocado, peeled and cubed
- 1/2 cup fresh cilantro leaves
- 3 tablespoon lime juice
- 1/2 teaspoon onion powder
- 1/2 teaspoon garlic powder
- 1/2 teaspoon chipotle hot pepper sauce
- 1/4 teaspoon salt
- 1/4 teaspoon ground cumin
- Baked tortilla chips

Directions:

1. Mix the first 9 ingredients in a food processor, then cover and blend until smooth. Serve along with chips.

Nutrition: Calories 85 Fat 4 Carbs 13 Protein 6

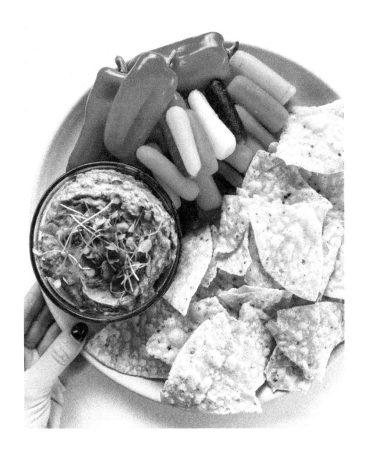

Crunchy Peanut Butter Apple Dip

Preparation Time: 10 minutes

Cooking Time: 10 minutes

Servings: 2

Ingredients:

- 1 carton (8 oz.) reduced-fat spreadable cream cheese
- 1 cup creamy peanut butter
- 1/4 cup fat-free milk
- 1 tablespoon brown sugar
- 1 teaspoon vanilla extract
- 1/2 cup chopped unsalted peanuts
- Apple slices

Directions:

1. Beat the initial 5 ingredients in a small bowl until combined. Mix in peanuts. Serve with slices of apple, then put the leftovers in the fridge.

Nutrition: Calories 125 Fat 5 Carbs 23 Protein 9

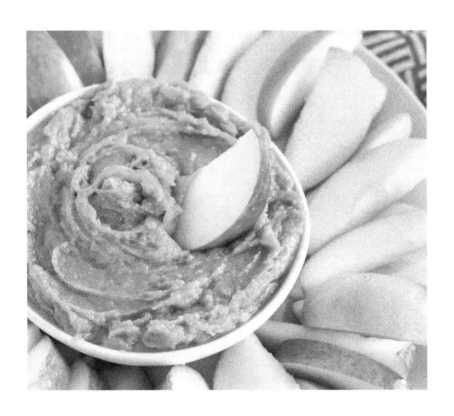

Herb Pockets

Preparation Time: 25 minutes

Cooking Time: 25 minutes

Servings: 3

Ingredients:

- 2/3 cup reduced-fat garlic-herb spreadable cheese
- 4 oz. reduced-fat cream cheese
- 2 tablespoon half-and-half cream
- 1 garlic clove, minced
- 1 tablespoon dried basil
- 1 teaspoon dried thyme
- 1/2 teaspoon celery salt
- 1/4 teaspoon dill weed
- 1/4 teaspoon salt
- 1/4 teaspoon pepper
- 3 to 4 drops hot pepper sauce
- 1/2 cup chopped canned water-packed artichoke hearts, rinsed and drained
- 1/4 cup chopped roasted red peppers
- 2 tubes (8 oz. each) refrigerated reduced-fat crescent rolls

Directions:

1. Beat garlic, cream, cream cheese, and spreadable cheese until blended in a small bowl. Beat in hot pepper sauce, pepper, salt, and herbs. Fold in red peppers and artichokes. Refrigerate, covered, for at least an hour.

2. Unroll both crescent roll dough tubes. Form every dough tube to a long rectangle on a lightly floured surface. Seal perforations and seams. Roll each to a 16x12-in. rectangle. Cut to 4 strips, lengthwise and 3 strips, width wise. Separate squares.

3. In the middle of each square, put 1 rounded tablespoon filling. Fold into half, making triangles. Seal by crimping edges. Trim if needed. Put onto ungreased baking sheets. Bake for 10-15 minutes or until golden brown at 375 degrees F. Serve warm.

Nutrition: Calories 245 Fat 5 Carbs 10 Protein 7

Creamy Cucumber Yogurt Dip

Preparation Time: 15 minutes

Cooking Time: 15 minutes

Servings: 4

Ingredients:

- 1 cup (8 oz.) reduced-fat plain yogurt
- 4 oz. reduced-fat cream cheese
- 1/2 cup chopped seeded peeled cucumber
- 1-1/2 teaspoon. finely chopped onion
- 1-1/2 teaspoon. snipped fresh dill or 1/2 teaspoon dill weed
- 1 teaspoon lemon juice
- 1 teaspoon grated lemon peel
- 1 garlic clove, minced
- 1/4 teaspoon salt
- 1/4 teaspoon pepper
- Assorted fresh vegetables

Directions:

1. Mix the cream cheese and yogurt in a small bowl. Stir in pepper, salt, garlic, peel, lemon juice, dill, onion, and cucumber. Put on the

cover and let it chill in the fridge. Serve it with the veggies.

Nutrition: Calories 55 Fat 4 Carbs 12 Protein 6

Chunky Cucumber Salsa

Preparation Time: 20 minutes

Cooking Time: 20 minutes

Servings: 4

Ingredients:

- 3 medium cucumbers, peeled and coarsely chopped
- 1 medium mango, coarsely chopped
- 1 cup frozen corn, thawed
- 1 medium sweet red pepper, coarsely chopped
- 1 small red onion, coarsely chopped
- 1 jalapeno pepper, finely chopped
- 3 garlic cloves, minced
- 2 tablespoon white wine vinegar
- 1 tablespoon minced fresh cilantro
- 1 teaspoon salt
- 1/2 teaspoon sugar
- 1/4 to 1/2 teaspoon cayenne pepper

Directions:

1. Mix all ingredients in a big bowl, then chill, covered, about 2 to 3 hours before serving.

Nutrition: Calories 215 Fat 5 Carbs 23 Protein 10

Healthier Guacamole

Preparation Time: 10 minutes

Cooking Time: 10 minutes

Servings: 4

Ingredients:

- 3/4 cup crumbled tofu
- 2 avocados - peeled and pitted, divided
- 1 teaspoon salt
- 1 teaspoon minced garlic
- 1 pinch cayenne pepper (optional)

Directions:

1. Prepare a food processor then put one avocado and tofu in it then blend well until it becomes smooth. Combine salt, lime juice, and the left avocado in a bowl.
2. Add in the garlic, tomatoes, cilantro, onion, and tofu-avocado mixture. Put in cayenne pepper.
3. Let it chill in the refrigerator for 1 hour to enhance the flavor or you can serve it right away.

Nutrition: Calories 534 Fat 5 Carbs 23 Protein 11

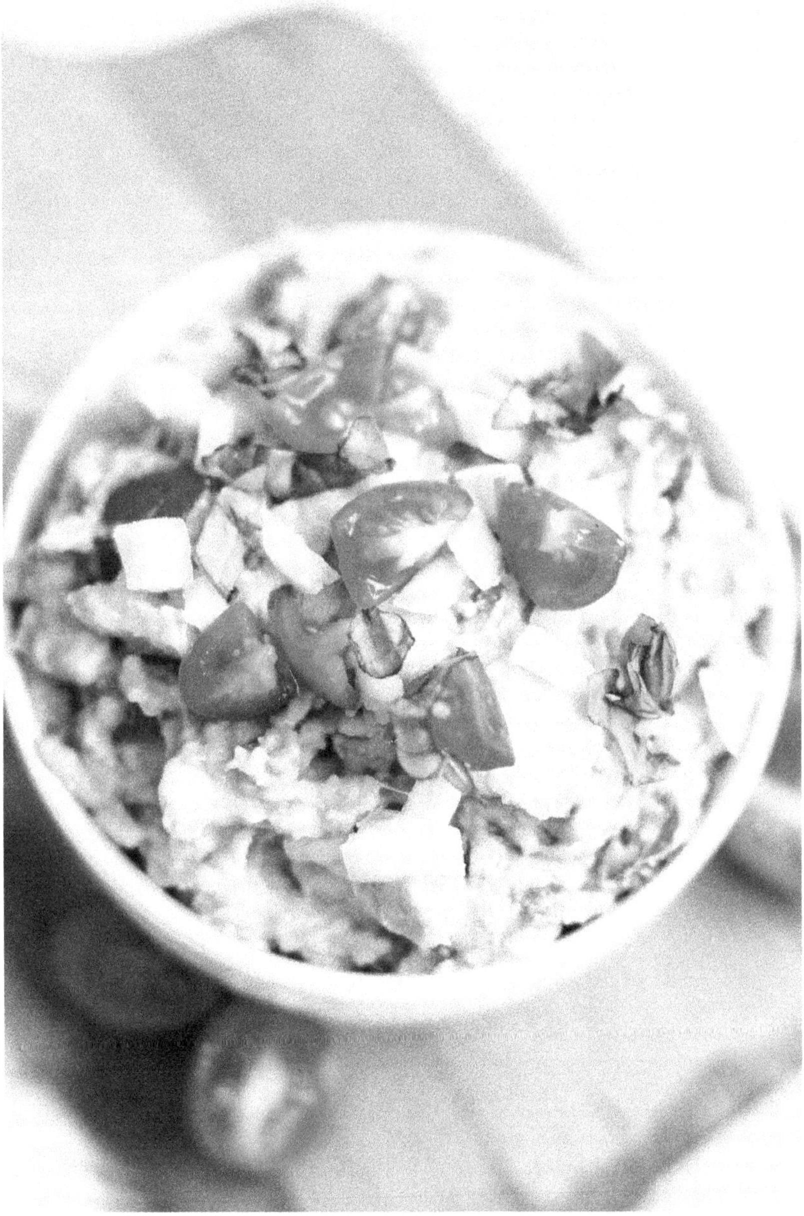

Garlic White Bean Dip

Preparation Time: 15 minutes

Cooking Time: 15 minutes

Servings: 2

Ingredients:

- 1/4 cup soft bread crumbs
- 2 tablespoon dry white wine or water
- 2 tablespoon olive oil
- 2 tablespoon lemon juice
- 4-1/2 teaspoon. minced fresh parsley
- 3 garlic cloves, peeled and halved
- 1/2 teaspoon salt
- 1/2 teaspoon snipped fresh dill or 1/4 teaspoon dill weed
- 1/8 teaspoon cayenne pepper
- Assorted fresh vegetables

Directions:

1. Mix wine and bread crumbs in a small bowl. Mix cayenne, dill, salt, garlic, parsley, beans, lemon juice, and oil in a food processor, then cover and blend until smooth.

2. Put in bread crumb mixture and process until well combined. Serve together with vegetables.

Nutrition: Calories 105 Fat 5 Carbs 12 Protein 6

Fruit Skewers

Preparation Time: 20 minutes

Cooking Time: 20 minutes

Servings: 2

Ingredients:

- cream cheese
- fat sour cream
- lime juice
- honey
- 1/2 teaspoon ground ginger
- 2 cups green grapes
- 2 cups fresh or canned unsweetened pineapple chunks
- 2 large red apples, cut into 1-inch pieces

Directions:

1. To make the dip, beat the sour cream and cream cheese in a small bowl until it becomes smooth. Beat in the ginger, honey, and lime juice until it becomes smooth.

2. Put the cover and let it chill in the fridge for a minimum of 1 hour.

3. Alternately thread the apples, pineapple, and grapes on 8 12-inch skewers. Serve it right away with the dip.

Nutrition: Calories 180 Fat 5 Carbs 28 Protein 4

Low-fat Stuffed Mushrooms

Preparation Time: 20 minutes

Cooking Time: 25 minutes

Servings: 6

Ingredients:

- 1 lb. large fresh mushrooms
- 3 tablespoons seasoned bread crumbs
- 3 tablespoons fat-free sour cream
- 2 tablespoons grated Parmesan cheese
- 2 tablespoons minced chives
- 2 tablespoons reduced-fat mayonnaise
- 2 teaspoons balsamic vinegar
- 2 to 3 drops hot pepper sauce, optional

Directions:

1. Take out the stems from the mushrooms, then put the cups aside. Chop the stems and set aside 1/3 cup (get rid of the leftover stems or reserve for later use).

2. Mix the reserved mushroom stems, hot pepper sauce if preferred, vinegar, mayonnaise, chives,

Parmesan cheese, sour cream, and breadcrumbs in a bowl, then stir well.

3. Put the mushroom caps on a cooking spray-coated baking tray and stuff it with the crumb mixture.

4. Let it boil for 5 to 7 minutes, placed 4-6 inches from the heat source, or until it turns light brown.

Nutrition: Calories 435 Fat 4 Carbs 23 Protein 9

Marinated Mushrooms

Preparation Time: 15 minutes

Cooking Time: 25 minutes

Servings: 8

Ingredients:

- 1 cup red wine
- 1/2 cup red wine vinegar
- 1/3 cup olive oil
- 2 tablespoon brown sugar
- 2 cloves garlic, minced
- 1 teaspoon crushed red pepper flakes
- 1/4 cup red bell pepper, diced
- 1 lb. small fresh mushrooms, washed and trimmed
- 1/4 cup chopped green onions
- 1/4 teaspoon dried oregano
- 1/2 teaspoon salt
- 1/4 teaspoon ground black pepper

Directions:

1. Mix the mushrooms, red pepper flakes, bell pepper, garlic, sugar, oil, vinegar, and wine in a saucepan on medium heat, then boil.

2. Put the cover and put it aside to let it cool.

3. Mix in pepper, salt, oregano, and green onions once cooled. Serve it at room temperature or chilled.

Nutrition: Calories 135 Fat 5 Carbs 13 Protein 8

Pumpkin Spice Spread

Preparation Time: 10 minutes

Cooking Time: 10 minutes

Servings: 4

Ingredients:

- 1 package (8 oz.) fat-free cream cheese
- 1/2 cup canned pumpkin
- Sugar substitute equivalent to 1/2 cup sugar
- 1 teaspoon ground cinnamon
- 1 teaspoon vanilla extract
- 1 teaspoon maple flavoring
- 1/2 teaspoon pumpkin pie spice
- 1/2 teaspoon ground nutmeg
- 1 carton (8 oz.) frozen reduced-fat whipped topping, thawed

Directions:

1. Mix well together sugar substitute, pumpkin, and cream cheese in a big bowl. Beat in nutmeg, pumpkin pie spice, maple flavoring, vanilla, and cinnamon.

2. Fold in whipped topping and chill until serving.

Nutrition: Calories 177 Fat 6 Carbs 21 Protein 11

Maple Bagel Spread

Preparation Time: 10 minutes

Cooking Time: 10 minutes

Servings: 1

Ingredients:

- cream cheese
- maple syrup
- cinnamon
- walnuts

Directions:

1. Beat the cinnamon, syrup, and cream cheese in a big bowl until it becomes smooth, then mix in walnuts.
2. Let it chill until ready to serve. Serve it with bagels.

Nutrition: Calories 586 Fat 7 Carbs 23 Protein 4

Italian Stuffed Artichokes

Preparation Time: 20 minutes

Cooking Time: 25 minutes

Servings: 4

Ingredients:

- 4 large artichokes
- 2 teaspoon lemon juice
- 2 cups soft Italian bread crumbs, toasted
- 1/2 cup grated Parmigiano-Reggiano cheese
- 1/2 cup minced fresh parsley
- 2 teaspoon Italian seasoning
- 1 teaspoon grated lemon peel
- 1/2 teaspoon pepper
- 1/4 teaspoon salt
- 1 tablespoon olive oil

Directions:

1. Level the bottom of each artichoke using a sharp knife and trim off 1-inch from the tops. Snip off tips of outer leaves using kitchen scissors, then brush lemon juice on cut edges. In a Dutch oven, stand the artichokes and pour 1-inch of

water, then boil. Lower the heat, put the cover, and let it simmer for 5 minutes or until the leaves near the middle pull out effortlessly.

2. Turn the artichokes upside down to drain. Allow it to stand for 10 minutes. Carefully scrape out the fuzzy middle part of the artichokes using a spoon and get rid of it.

3. Mix the salt, pepper, lemon peel, Italian seasoning, garlic, parsley, cheese, and breadcrumbs in a small bowl, then add olive oil and stir well. Gently spread the artichoke leaves apart, then fill it with breadcrumb mixture.

4. Put it in a cooking spray-coated 11x7-inch baking dish. Let it bake for 10 minutes at 350 degrees F without cover, or until the filling turns light brown.

Nutrition: Calories 543 Fat 5 Carbs 44 Protein 6

Enchilada sauce

Preparation Time: 10 minutes

Cooking Time: 10 minutes

Servings: 13

Ingredients:

- 1½ tablespoon MCT oil
- ½ tablespoon chili powder
- ½ tablespoon whole wheat flour
- ½ teaspoon ground cumin
- ¼ teaspoon oregano (dried or fresh)
- ¼ teaspoon salt (or to taste)
- 1 garlic clove (minced)
- 1 tablespoon tomato paste
- 1 cup vegetable broth
- ½ teaspoon apple vinegar
- ½ teaspoon ground black pepper

Directions:

1. Heat a small saucepan over medium heat.
2. Add the MCT oil and minced garlic to the pan and sauté for about 1 minute.

3. Mix the dry spices and flour in a medium bowl and pour the dry mixture into the saucepan.
4. Stir in the tomato paste immediately, and slowly pour in the vegetable broth, making sure that everything combines well.
5. When everything is mixed thoroughly, bring up the heat to medium-high until it gets to a simmer and cook for about 3 minutes or until the sauce becomes a bit thicker.
6. Remove the pan from the heat and add the vinegar with the black pepper, adding more salt and pepper to taste.

Nutrition: Calories 225 Fat 4 Carbs 33 Protein 5

Conclusion

Vegan recipes do not need to be boring. There are so many different combinations of veggies, fruits, whole grains, beans, seeds, and nuts that you will be able to make unique meal plans for many months. These recipes contain the instructions along with the necessary ingredients and nutritional information.

If you ever come across someone complaining that they can't follow the plant-based diet because it's expensive, hard to cater for, lacking in variety, or tasteless, feel free to have them take a look at this book. In no time, you'll have another companion walking beside you on this road to healthier eating and better living.

Although healthy, many people are still hesitant to give vegan food a try. They mistakenly believe that these would be boring, tasteless, and complicated to make. This is the farthest thing from the truth.

Fruits and vegetables are organically delicious, fragrant, and vibrantly colored. If you add herbs, mushrooms, and nuts to the mix, dishes will always come out packed full of flavor it only takes a bit of effort and time to prepare great-tasting vegan meals for your family.

How easy was that? Don't we all want a seamless and easy way to cook like this?

I believe cooking is taking a better turn and the days, when we needed so many ingredients to provide a decent meal, were gone. Now, with easy tweaks, we can make delicious, quick, and easy meals. Most importantly, we get to save a bunch of cash on groceries.

I am grateful for downloading this book and taking the time to read it. I know that you have learned a lot and you had a great time reading it. Writing books is the best way to share the skills I have with your and the best tips too.

I know that there are many books and choosing my book is amazing. I am thankful that you stopped and took time to decide. You made a great decision and I am sure that you enjoyed it.

I will be even happier if you will add some comments. Feedbacks helped by growing and they still do. They help me to choose better content and new ideas. So, maybe your feedback can trigger an idea for my next book.

Hopefully, this book has helped you understand that vegetarian recipes and diet can improve your life, not only by improving your health and helping you lose weight, but also by saving you money and time. I sincerely hope that the recipes provided in this book have proven to be quick, easy, and delicious, and have provided you with enough variety to keep your taste buds interested and curious.

I hope you enjoyed reading about my book!

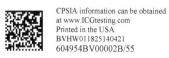

CPSIA information can be obtained
at www.ICGtesting.com
Printed in the USA
BVHW011825140421
604954BV00002B/55

9 781801 835602